Three Bowl Diet

To order additional copies, please contact us.
BookSurge, LLC
www.booksurge.com
1-866-308-6235
orders@booksurge.com

Three Bowl Diet

The Key to Weight Control Forever

Keith N. Haley

Imprint Productions
2005

Three Bowl Diet

CONTENTS

The Three Bowl Diet Is Dedicated To All Those Worthy Souls Who Have Struggled With Weight Control.

CHAPTER I

INTRODUCTION

Let's start by taking this test. Look down at your stomach. Is it too big? Can you see your toes? If seeing your toes makes you feel good, then grab those love handles just above your hips. Do you really think your life's soul mate wants to see those ghastly things for the duration?

These were the static tests. If you can't see your toes because your stomach is in the way or your love handles quiver when you breathe, you got an "F" on the static test.

Maybe you will do better on the mobility test. You can do it indoors or outdoors. Walk 20 steps briskly across the room, across the street, or down the sidewalk. Do you feel anything shaking around your waist, hips, or thighs? If you do, you just got an "F" on the mobility test.

You probably knew before you started you would flunk both of these tests. Don't feel too bad, half of America would flunk them. In fact, let's get real, you are FAT! You and I have probably gone from diet to diet, weight loss to weight gain for years, maybe decades, and you are at the point of giving up.

But now is the time to get down on your hand and knees and thank your Creator you found this book. Then jump up and shout "Halleluiah, I have found it!" Success is just around the corner. Don't go buy new clothes yet, but you can start shopping. The Three Bowl Diet is here!

✵✵✵

SO WHAT'S WRONG WITH OTHER DIETS?

We are glad you asked. Have you tried other diets? We know the answer to that and not one of them worked to the point of your losing weight and keeping it off. These diets are hard to follow for a lot reasons. Let's look at some.

Counting Calories

Some of these diets want you to count calories. Really! Counting and math are hard enough, but it's near impossible to count calories when you can't even see them, right? Have you ever seen a calorie? Neither has anyone else. Plus, counting calories is BORING!

Counting the Steps You Take Each Day

Another diet plan, plus exercise, wants you to count how many steps you take in a day's time. Are you kidding me? It is hard enough to count pocket change let alone 10,000-14,000 steps a day. This program is from the Amish, but we all know that growing and harvesting food, eating, and counting their steps are about the only things they are allowed to do that aren't sinful. No offense, but NO THANKS!

Counting Bites of Food

A recent diet wants you to count the bites of food you eat each day and restricts you to 75 bites each day. We are not kidding. How can that work? We all know people who could woof down a small pan pizza, a double Whopper, or a KFC chicken breast in one big bite. You don't lost weight that way. Plus, you know when we get to counting above 20, we lose our place anyway and have to start over. In addition, what we try to count again is already in our belly.

Measuring and Weighing Food

This is one of the kookiest of all the diet plans. They want you to measure and weigh all of the food you are going to eat in order to not get fat. You have to be kidding me! Who is going to carry a measuring cup and scale to TGIF's on a Friday night out for dinner? I think we can sum this diet up like this: MEASURING + COUNTING = DOUBLE BORING! You see, I am not totally against math.

Food Restrictions

Finally, you have the myriad of food restriction diets for weight loss and health: no meat; no sugar; no starch; no carbohydrates; no cholesterol; no protein; etc., etc. The only tangible thing you are going to accomplish with this diet, aside from never tasting anything good, is to put all of the farmers and ranchers out of work. Who wants to live with that kind of guilt besides a few thousand PETA members?

***

THE NUTS AND BOLTS OF THE THREE BOWL DIET

OK, what is this diet all about? Enough of the prelims! This diet is so simple and effective. Here are the details:

1. The Three Bowl Diet requires no counting above the number "3," I promise.
2. You do not have to measure anything beyond making sure your bowl is filled to the brim. Anyone can do that with the naked eye.
3. You do have to purchase 3 bowls. If you are short on cash, you can use the same bowl three times in the same day. I would, however, suggest washing it out carefully between meals.
4. While we will suggest putting some very specific food items in each of the bowls, you do not have to. How is that for an easy-to-follow diet? Eat what you want.
5. THE BIG POINT: You fill your bowl with food to the brim (not beyond), three times a day, with any

food you want, and keep doing that until you reach your desired weight. That is simple enough that even a member of Congress or a Ph.D. could understand it. Wait a minute, maybe not a Ph.D., they have to make things complicated.

In the few chapters that follow, I will describe the Three Bowl Diet plan and then you can be on your way to a slimmer life.

CHAPTER 2

BOWL NUMBER ONE – BREAKFAST

Everyone knows how important breakfast is. Well, at least almost everyone does. If you are not accustomed to eating breakfast, you need to start. Think about it. You have probably not eaten since the previous evening meal unless you woofed down a giant bag of Fritos and a small pizza while gawking at TV after dinner.

Having not eaten for so long means your body is sort of "out of fuel" at this point and breakfast is your first stop at the "filling station" for the day ahead. Plus, you never know, eating breakfast may improve your disposition if you are a morning grump.

***

WHAT DO I PUT IN BOWL NUMBER ONE?

Since this is your first bowl on the first day of the Three Bowl Diet, what you put in the bowl is important. But you know, it is not that important. After all you could almost live on eating the box for a Quarter Pounder and a few crackers, but let's don't try that.

Three general rules apply to filling the bowls during the day.

I. You only eat, no matter what, three level bowls full of food each day. No exceptions!

2. Fill the bowl with food that would be appropriate for that meal. For breakfast you could fill the bowl with scrambled eggs, sausage, and even a small slice of bread. You may want fruit. That is OK too. It all goes in the same bowl since the food all goes to the same place anyway.

3. Hold on, here we contradict rule two. Fill the bowl at breakfast, or at any other meal, with whatever you want to eat even if it is not ordinarily eaten at that particular meal you are preparing. If you like apple pie, go for it. Fill the bowl to the rim, but no higher. Place a sheet of paper over the top of the bowl and make sure the food does not extend beyond the rim. If it does, level it! Remember, you are trying to lose weight.

Could you have pizza for breakfast? You bet you could! You could have it three days in a row if you want to. But recall those healthy food groups? Try to eat some of each. Eventually you will grow tired of eating the same thing all of the time anyway, so we know you will get a "balanced diet."

Finally, the food can be hot or cold. It is your choice and it makes no difference, but steak tastes a lot better cooked than raw. If you prefer it raw, you may not be that far away in your family lineage from creatures that move on all fours!

Eat slowly, be sure to chew thoroughly, and enjoy breakfast.

CHAPTER 3

BOWL NUMBER 2 – LUNCH

OK, notice that you have not been doing a lot of counting or high math. But it is lunch time and you are ready for Bowl Number 2. This is still single digit math so I know you are with us. Just think if you were counting calories or, even worse, bites, you would already be lost unless you are an accountant, engineer, or math teacher.

But let's face it now. Bowl Number 2 is likely to present a problem that I know you can solve. I did, so I know you can.

We start this chapter with a quiz. Where do we usually eat lunch unless it is the weekend? OK, if you can't guess, here is the answer: "Outside our home."

Now you are confronted with a dilemma. I am eating with my regular lunch buddies at Ruby Tuesday's or Aunt Polly's Home Cookin' Spot. Do I whip out my bowl and set it on the table? You could, but Aunt Polly might accuse you of stealing dishes when you put the bowl back into your overcoat pocket when it is time to leave. It would show, however, THREE BOWL DIET commitment to carry it with you! You have allies all over America. Don't forget that.

Solution # 1 is to order a bowl of soup, some chili, or a side salad and your bowl is filled and your problem is solved. Eat the contents.

Solution # 2 is to ask for an empty soup bowl with whatever you order, and do the measuring of your order after the server brings it. The server will think that you are a bit odd, but they see worse. What if a guy on a diet came in with scales and measuring cups just before you? Get my point.

Solution # 3 is a bit mystical and you may gain followers from just performing this ritual. Keep in mind, people really love kooks. Freak is really in now. After you receive your order at the table (a hotdog, French fries, lasagna, prunes, or whatever), close your eyes for a minute or two and try to get an image in your mind of exactly what your bowl looks like, height, radius, circumference (duh, can you picture that?). Then when you open your eyes, provided you did not fall asleep, use your fork to accumulate on one side of your plate the exact amount of the food you ordered that would have filled your bowl to the brim. Problem solved. Eat only that amount of the food from your plate and ask for a doggy bag for the rest or push it off on your friends.

Of course, you should try to order what will fit in your Bowl Number 2, and this usually means you eliminate the trucker's rack of ribs special and a large pizza. I am sure you get the idea. In a way, it is a better intelligence test than those shrinks give, trying to get you to put square pegs in round holes. They can always do it the right way since they bought the test and practiced ahead of time. Anyway, I am sure you can match your order and bowl size with a little practice.

Remember, if the order is too big for the bowl, you can always share it with your lunch buddies, or take the extra food home for Fido.

Enjoy your meal, chew your food thoroughly, and enjoy the company of your friends and they will see already that you have more time to talk at lunch.

One more meal to go and you will have completed the whole Three Bowl Diet cycle. You won't be hungry, well I mean really hungry, and you won't be cutting out any of those good things you like. I mean you could have had an ice cream lunch, right?

CHAPTER 4

BOWL NUMBER THREE - DINNER

As they say in Texas, "you done good" so far! You have gotten through two meals already, gained the admiration of your lunch table server who now thinks you are some sort of mystic, and have come to the point of eating your last meal of the day. Supper is really a breeze! You are more than likely back home where you can rely on your bowl to determine how much you eat for this third and last meal of the day.

Now the only thing that can set you off at supper time, short of a hunger attack, is a telephone solicitor calling just when you are ready to eat. One of two quick lines here will work: (1) Tell the caller you just filed bankruptcy or (2) that you are having a wake at your house at the moment. The solicitor will hang up before you can!

I should point out one more thing. Notice that you have not counted above two at this point. Imagine if you were on one of those other diets. By now you would have counted up into the thousands. It is not that I'm against math, but unnecessary counting is boring.

***

DINNER GUESTS
One possible unique problem exists at dinner. You are go-

ing to have dinner guests and more than likely they are members of your family. If some or all of them joined you at breakfast, they probably didn't have much to say, since most people don't talk in the morning. But now they are all warmed up and awake, and they might be in the mood to give you a little razing. But by now you are invincible. You have already won two battles at the table today and you're not likely to throw in the towel at dinner.

I think you need a few attack lines that you can use on them to keep them from bothering you. Try this one first. Pick on someone your own size. This will work particularly well if you are substantially heavier than they are. If that doesn't work, tell them that you will have to remove them from the table. Since you are likely to be larger than they are, that should not be too much trouble. Next, you may have to tell them that you will remove your "exalted presence" from their company, and it will be their loss for sure. Then you could try this. You could appeal to their aesthetic qualities. Tell them how much more they will enjoy you when your body compares closely to a television model. Emphasize how much they will want to be around you when look like that.

OK, you may have to resort to a Texas solution. Turn the dinner table over and dump the food in their laps. I do emphasize that this is a last resort, but there is no doubt they will get the message. Of course, you may be eating alone after that, but sometimes that can't be all bad.

✳✳✳

THE FOOD

You have one more bowl to fill today, so let's get to it. Actually, this should be your best meal. First of all, here you are with family, and they should be supportive. Secondly, you can catch up on family business. Good conversation at the dinner table is at least half of the value of having dinner with your family. This meal also provides you with the greatest variety of food choices as dinners often do.

Another thing that you want to remember is who cares what they're having for dinner, because you're going to get a little of all of it anyway. Nothing is restricted from your diet other than possibly the excessive intake of spinach. Popeye is the only character who can survive that!

Look carefully over the serving platters and bowls that are on the table and think about what you want to eat. The only restriction you have is to be sure that the total contents of your bowl do not extend above the brim. That means for example, that you can have spaghetti, lamb chops, apple pie, ice cream, or any other darn thing you want.

I suppose there is this other benefit. Because you are not chewing and eating as much, you will have more time to talk with your family. That is not all bad. If you happen to have a kid or two you can't stand, you might actually end up liking them since you talk with them more at the dinner table.

***

TAKING STOCK

Let's sum up what you've been through today.

1. For the first time in maybe months you did not eat like a pig!

2. You ate only three bowls of food filled with whatever you wanted to put in them. No food restrictions on this diet. Remember, you cannot maintain your current body weight eating only three bowls of food each day no matter what you put in the bowl.

3. You friends and family admire your courage and deter-

mination for starting another diet, or they think you are nuts for buying a diet book that contains so few pages and whose diet is so simple to follow. The author thanks you!

4. You have developed some discipline and fortitude for the days ahead. You have been victorious 3 times already today, and tomorrow all you have to do is the same thing. Past performance predicts future behavior. Your future "looks" great.

In the final chapter I offer some tips for the completion of your Three Bowl Diet and the days beyond.

CHAPTER 5

THE GLORIOUS ROAD AHEAD

In this last chapter, I only have one objective. That is to see that you get some encouragement for the glorious road that lies ahead. I have no doubt that if you persist, you will succeed. Remember that you may fail 1000 times, but you only have to succeed once. YOU CAN DO IT!

Okay, I suppose this is the time to confess that I tricked you. But I'm not ashamed because it was all for a good reason. You have learned to eat proper portions at meal time. Isn't that the real secret to weight control? You simply have to not overeat. By using the three bowls, you learned to select and eat a reasonable amount of food at each meal. The bowl was your teacher! Cherish the bowl, preserve the bowl, and worship the bowl, because it brought you to a point that you've never been to before. Your weight will soon be in the normal range, and you have the formula for staying there your entire life.

Nevertheless, you need to take one day at a time. Keeping weight off by eating proper portions is a struggle at every meal. Temptation exists at every turn. Yet even those succulent and addictive foods can be sampled and enjoy if you remember the secret of the three bowls. Fill the bowl to the brim with whatever you like, but be cautious about second helpings and heavy snacks between meals. Remember, you will persist until you succeed!

Now even though your weight is not under control having been on the Three Bowl Diet only one day, you do have your appetite under control already. But below are a few things that you can do that will assist you in maintaining confidence and in controlling your weight.

I. Get a mirror. It's important. While being the correct weight will make you feel good, let's not kid ourselves, you also wanted to look good. Looking good means you have to study yourself and that requires a certain amount of detail. A mirror will tell you no lies. Look at yourself often in the mirror as you participate in the Three Bowl Diet. In a matter of time, you'll notice a physical change in your body. Your hips will slim, your waist will narrow, and your thighs will no longer rub between your legs.

2. Dress up once in awhile. America needs it. We've come to a point where casual is almost depressing in clothes. Personally, if I see one more pair of cargo pants topped by a baggy T-shirt, worn by an unwashed and unshaved mutant, I think I will puke.

That beautiful body that you now possess or that you are on the way to possessing should be properly adorned once in awhile at least. If you don't own one good set of clothes, go purchase an outfit. Wear the clothes somewhere in your new body and enjoy the compliments that people will pay you. You owe it to yourself to do this. You know what? You can even buy some good-looking underwear and look at yourself in the mirror. You'll appreciate your new look for sure. While you're at it, woman or man, get a new hairstyle, since it's a new you anyway, you might as well top it off appropriately.

3. Weigh yourself every day. A lot of diet commentators do not want you to do this. Don't believe them. This whole thing is about weight isn't it? Then keep a record of your weight every

day. Put it in a small notebook and look back at it once in while, and you'll be amazed at the progress you have made. That "look back" will be motivating. If you happen to gain a few pounds, and don't do anything about it right away, you can look at the record book and recall the progress you made when you started the three bowl diet and realize that if you lost that much weight, taking off a few extra pounds will be no problem at all. You know the secret. It's in the bowls!

4. Don't eat late in the evening if you can avoid it. It loads you down with calories that you don't expend by walking around and doing the normal things that you do during the day. Sometimes this is not convenient, but most of the time you can avoid it. Try walking about a half hour or so after meals if you can. It is an old boxer's trick to never let a meal lie in your stomach without some later movement.

5. With all of the humility you can conjure up be proud of your new body! You worked very hard to get it.

6. Don't forget prayer when you need help. It works!

Above all, PERSIST UNTIL YOU SUCCEED! A journey of 1000 miles begins with a single step. At the end of the first day of the three bowl diet you have started that journey and you are on your way to success.

Maybe you can start your own classes on the Three Bowl Diet. You can be the seminar leader and make some money by teaching others the secret of the three bowls. Of course, every class needs a textbook, so please contact me and I will be glad to supply them at a group price rate. So far I have not made enough money on this book to pay for one good night out. Any help you can give me will be appreciated. Oprah Winfrey hasn't called either, but I have a suit pressed and my shoes are shined, so I'm ready to go at a moment's notice.

If you become successful using the Three Bowl Diet, drop

me a line and let me know how well you did. If you didn't, don't bother to tell me, but maybe you can sell the book on eBay and recover your loss. Just kidding, I know you're going to be successful.

Best of luck. Remember, Three Bowl Dieters all over the world are behind you! You cannot and will not fail.

ABOUT THE AUTHOR

Keith Haley is a Professor of Criminal Justice, teaching in both graduate and undergraduate degree programs. He has also served as an Associate Vice President for Special Projects at Tiffin University. Mr. Haley has also been the Dean of the School of Criminal Justice, and the Dean of the School of Off-Campus Learning at Tiffin University and has acted as the primary contact for the TU MBA program in Bucharest, Romania and was the head of the Tiffin University Romania Study team that worked to establish a Master of Community Justice Administration degree program at the University of Bucharest, one of Europe's oldest and most influential universities. This program has now had 4 graduating classes of Romanian justice professionals.

He has also served in the following positions: Coordinator of the Criminal Justice Programs at Collin County Community College in Texas with academic programs at three campuses; Executive Director of the Ohio Peace Officer Standards and Training Commission, the state's law enforcement standards and training agency, certifying more than two dozen professional positions in law enforcement, corrections, and private security, including all police recruits in Ohio; Chairman of the Criminal Justice Program at the University of Cincinnati which offered B.S. and M.S. degrees in criminal justice; police officer in Dayton, Ohio; Community School Director in Springfield, Ohio; Director of the Criminal Justice Program at Redlands Community College in Oklahoma; electronics repairman and NCO in the U.S. Marines.

Haley holds the following degrees: B.S. in Education from Wright State University; M.S. in Criminal Justice from Michigan State University.

Haley is the author, co-author, and/or editor of 16 books including revised editions and several self-published books, one of which has sold internationally, several book chapters, many articles in criminal justice trade and other kinds of periodical publications, and papers, and has served as a consultant to many public service, university, business, and industrial organizations on management, online learning, criminal justice research, and memory skills for many different kinds of professionals.

The American Association of University Administrators presented the 2001 Nikolai N. Khaladjan International Award for Innovation in Higher Education to Haley for his leadership in the Tiffin University/University of Bucharest "Partnership for Justice" project which established a graduate school of criminal justice administration in Bucharest, Romania that is now being replicated in other universities in that nation. The Khaladjan Award is given to the higher education program that is the most innovative and has the widest potential for impact on post-secondary education.

Mr. Haley's research interests are varied. He has published works on criminal justice management and supervision, police human resources management, the administration of justice, job-hunting skills, memory skills, the applications of the World Wide Web and the Internet to law enforcement and corrections, online learning and teaching, crime analysis, firearms in America, gangster rap and culture, campus policing, police academy management, crime and justice in Texas and Ohio, and education and training in criminal justice. Haley is also co-author with Robert Bohm of *Introduction to Criminal Justice 4th Edition 2005, McGraw-Hill*, one of the more widely used introductory criminal justice texts in colleges and universities. The book has been translated into the Romanian language under the title Justitia Penala (Professor Theodora Ene, University of Bucharest, Translator) as was reviewed and approved by Professor General Pavel Abraham, Secretary of State in the Ministry of the Interior, and is used in a graduate program for criminal justice leaders in Romania at the University of Bucharest.

Haley is also the author, coauthor, or editor of the following books: *With Liberty and Guns for All: A Primer on America's Firearms Debate; Crime Analysis Issues, Applications and Techniques; Critical Issues in Campus Policing; Crime and Punishment in the Lone Star State; Texas Crime, Texas Justice; Ohio Crime, Ohio Justice.* International issues in criminal justice are also current research interests for Mr. Haley.

Mr. Haley has conducted memory seminars for many police agencies, large corporations such as Procter and Gamble, General Electric, and Cincinnati Milacron, school districts, colleges and universities, and other private and public service organizations.